Teaching Beauty
Leadership Skills for Educators

Christa McDearmon

ISBN: 1494448424
ISBN-13: 9781494448424

DEDICATION

To all those dedicated to making the world a more
beautiful place.
One licensed professional at a time.

And Maxine Maughan-
who taught me too many things to list.

CONTENTS

I- Integrity is the most valuable form of currency.

J- Juggling is for clowns.

K- Kindness in everything.

L- Love yourself, a lot.

M- Money making is their goal.

N- No is an okay word.

O- Observe.

P- Please and Thank You.

Q- Question Everything.

R- Remove yourself from the situation.

S- Surrender your ego.

T- Try again.

U - Understand Nothing.

V - Value everything.

W - Write it down or it didn't happen.

X - X marks the spot.

Y - Why am I doing this again?

Z - Zen. Find your peace at the end of each day.

FORWARD

This manual was developed specifically with the cosmetology school and educator in mind.
Although these skills can be life changing for anyone wanting to develop their own unique leadership identity.

As an owner, educator, or instructor, do you feel as if you've been placed in a leadership role without any formal training, or specific education to help you navigate this role? This can wreak havoc in our cosmetology schools, as I'm sure many of you can attest to.

What is wonderful about our industry is that because we all face the same challenges in our schools, we can unite and support each other in growing and developing our industry. Our focus should not have to be on managing the day-to-day trivial situations that seem to pop up continually, detracting from why we have chosen the path of becoming an educator. We are here to change lives! Each of us has what it takes to be an amazing leader. Yes, you! The one reading this and doubting your ability. The one who dreads stepping into your school and finding students out of dress code. Cell phones buzzing in the hallways. Soda spills and snack crumbs covering the classrooms. Eye-rolls of 8-week old students who already know more than you… It's time you've been given the skills and confidence to gain back control.

I'm going to share with you the ABC's of leadership. The more you immerse yourself and your school in these concepts the better your results will be. Take the time to think deeply about your personal leadership abilities and capabilities as you ponder this alphabet of new perspectives. You'll find the only person stopping you from becoming the leader you would like to be, is yourself.

Good luck on your journey. It's worth the walk.

THE ROAD NOT TAKEN

Two roads diverged in a yellow wood,
and sorry I could not travel both
and be one traveler, long I stood
and looked down one as far as I could
to where it bent in the undergrowth;

Then took the other, as just as fair,
and having perhaps the better claim
because it was grassy and wanted wear,
though as for that the passing there
had worn them really about the same,

And both that morning equally lay

in leaves no step had trodden black.

Oh, I kept the first for another day!

Yet knowing how way leads on to way

I doubted if I should ever come back.

I shall be telling this with a sigh

somewhere ages and ages hence:

Two roads diverged in a wood, and I,

I took the one less traveled by,

and that has made all the difference.

Robert Frost

JOURNALING

As we begin our leadership journey, you'll notice we've included journaling pages after each chapter. We don't want you to just read this book. We want you to actively participate in your journey. Reading alone is not going to make you a better leader or educator. So why journaling?

Scientific evidence supports that journaling provides unexpected benefits. The act of writing accesses your left brain, which is analytical and rational. While your left brain is occupied, your right brain is free to create, intuit and feel. In sum, writing removes mental blocks and allows you to use all of your brainpower to better understand yourself, others and the world around you. By journaling, you'll begin to experience these benefits:

Clarify your thoughts and feelings. Do you ever seem all jumbled up inside, unsure of what you want or feel? Taking a few minutes to jot down your thoughts and emotions (no editing!) will quickly get you in touch with your internal world.

Know yourself better. By writing routinely you will get to know what makes you feel happy and confident. You will also become clear about situations and people who are toxic for you — important information for your emotional well-being.

Reduce stress. Writing about anger, sadness and other painful emotions helps to release the intensity of these feelings. By doing so you will feel calmer and better able to stay in the present.

Solve problems more effectively. Typically we problem solve from a left-brained, analytical perspective. But sometimes the answer can only be found by engaging right-brained creativity and intuition. Writing unlocks these other capabilities, and affords the opportunity for unexpected solutions to seemingly unsolvable problems.

Resolve disagreements with others. Writing about misunderstandings rather than stewing over them will help you to understand another's point of view. And you just may come up with a sensible resolution to the conflict.

In addition to all of these wonderful benefits, keeping a journal allows you to track patterns, improvement, and growth over time. When current circumstances appear insurmountable, you will be able to look back on previous dilemmas that you have since resolved.

Purcell, M. (2006). The Health Benefits of

Journaling. *Psych Central.*

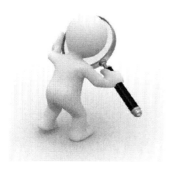

ACKNOWLEDGE IT TAKES HARD WORK TO BE GREAT

A dream doesn't become reality through magic; it takes sweat, determination and hard work.

Colin Powell

Picture your dream school, or your dream career as an educator. Looks good doesn't it? A big, beautiful school with clean floors, sparkling mirrors, organized rows of color tubes and perm rods, and bright shining faces lining up at the door, ready to absorb all of your hard work and dedication.

Now wake up and face reality!

This is hard work! Day in and day out it takes patience, persistence, desire, passion and compassion, strength of heart and mind, and more energy in a day than the average person finds in a week.

Be prepared to be emotionally knocked down, mentally numb and physically exhausted.

Are you thoroughly discouraged now? Wait, this hasn't been inspiring?

Here's the good news. It's worth it. You can acknowledge these feelings and still live the dream every morning of walking in your big, beautiful school with clean floors, sparkling mirrors, organized rows of color tubes and perm rods, and bright shining faces lining up at the door, ready to absorb all of your hard work and dedication.

Acknowledging it takes hard work to be great is an important first step in achieving your dream of a successful career. Are you ready to take the leap to becoming the best school, leader, and educator you can be?

Before moving through the next chapters, it's important to note that if you're not ready to become a leader, these exercises will not work for you. Change is not easy, and neither are some of these principles. If you find yourself saying these ideas are ridiculous and won't work in your school, take time to reflect on why you feel that way. You'll find at the root of your resistance is the fear of failure. It's easier to not change and blame your circumstance on your school, other staff members, the environment, or the area, than to take the leap and risk failing. To risk feeling stupid or outcast by your peers. To feel responsible to holding yourself or others more accountable. These are normal feelings. These are okay feelings. Remember you have a huge support system of other leaders that have been there, and I'll let you know how to build your amazing support system later. But let me tell you, it's a much better view from up here, so what are you waiting for? Let's make the climb together.

Before continuing, let's take a few moments to reflect why you've chosen this career path. Answer the following questions honestly with yourself. This is a personal exercise that will help you as we move through this manual.

Why did you decide to become an educator?

_____

_____

_____

List some strengths that you feel help you navigate your position.

_____

_____

_____

Do you feel like you have any weaknesses you cannot overcome? (Hint: No one has weaknesses they cannot overcome)

_____

_____

_____

What are some of your long term goals as it applies to your career. What have YOU done to help bring you closer to achieving your goals?

_____

_____

_____

Take a few minutes to envision your dream school and career. What does this look like to you?

_____

_____

_____

What are you doing now that does not match your vision?

_____

_____

_____

Who do you blame for your school, your students and yourself not operating the way that you would like?

_____

_____

_____

What are a few things you would change if you could? Whose responsibility is it to make these changes in your institution and culture?

_____

_____

_____

Do you feel like you have the skills it takes to be a leader in your school and in your industry?

_____

_____

_____

Are you open-minded and ready to try out new techniques that will propel you into a leadership role?

_____

_____

_____

Jot down any other thoughts that have popped in your head while answering these questions.

_____

_____

_____

Hold on to these answers as we'll be coming back to them throughout this manual.

LEADERSHIP JOURNAL

_____

_____

_____

_____

_____

_____

_____

_____

_____

_____

_____

_____

_____

_____

_____

_____

_____

_____

LEADERSHIP JOURNAL

_____

_____

_____

_____

_____

_____

_____

_____

_____

_____

_____

_____

_____

_____

_____

_____

_____

_____

_____

_____

_____

_____

_____

_____

B

BUILD A SOLID FOUNDATION TO STAND ON.

.

A successful man is one who can lay a firm foundation with the bricks others have thrown at him.

David Brinkley

It's wonderful to have a group of educators who all want to be great. But if we are all running around with individual dreams of success and different ideas of how to achieve our visions, this is a recipe for disaster.

In order to run a successful school or be a successful leader and educator you must have parameters.

Something solid to stand on and support you. These are called policies, systems and agreements.

Policies are essentially rules. These are standards we have in place so that the school runs smoothly and consistently. Your state board and government accreditation agencies have policies or rules in place that your school must follow in order to comply with state and federal laws. Your school may also place policies such as dress code standards and cell phone policies. These can vary from school to school. Did you know that once your school places a policy in writing in a handbook or contract that it becomes an accreditation (government) policy that you to comply with it?

Systems are how we do things. You should have a detailed and written system for everything from following your outlined curriculum to disciplinary policies. E.g. you get two written warnings for being late for school, the third time you will be suspended for <blank> amount of time. Or a no excuse policy on dress code- you will be clocked out and sent home to change. Period.

Agreements are what you make when you choose to work for your school. Agreements are what students make when they enroll in school. Agreements are what owners make when they open a school. Agreements state that you, your student's, the owner, and anyone else involved agree to follow the policies and systems while working at or attending the institution.

Everyone needs policies, systems and agreements in order to feel independent, confident and successful. Growing up as young children we made agreements with our parents that we wouldn't play with matches or talk to strangers. We had systems for checking our Halloween candy before eating it. As teens, we were taught the rules of the road and how to drive safely. As young adults, we attended cosmetology school and read our student handbook to ensure we showed up our first day in the right outfit. By having polices (rules) and systems in place, it allows us to feel safe, and secure. Once we feel these initial feelings of safety, it allows us more freedom and confidence to explore our new surroundings, careers and leadership skills without feeling the risk of failure.

So what are these policies, systems, and agreements? Well, you probably have a lot of them in place right now. Some you might not even be aware of. These come from regulatory agencies that tell us what governing laws apply to you. State agencies that regulate the practices you teach in your state. Fire evacuation plans and blood spill procedures. You have systems in your lesson plans that tell you what a 90 degree angle is and to properly process a color that's 50% grey. As an educator or instructor, you probably have an employee handbook that outlines your dress code, personal time off, employee expectations and other policies your establishment has in place. As a school, you also have a student handbook, these are the agreements put in place for your students to abide by. We are surrounded by systems.

Are you aware of the policies and systems your school has in place?

_____

_____

_____

What are some of the reoccurring issues facing your school? E.g. Cell phone or dress code policies. Do you have written policies on these? Why are you or aren't you following them?

_____

_____

_____

Do you have any unwritten policies? Policies that you enforce but are not found in your handbooks or contracts? Where did these come from?

_____

_____

_____

List as many systems as you can think of that are effective (or should be) in your school. This would be a great activity to brainstorm with your whole team.

_____

_____

_____

_____

_____

_____

Now again, being honest with yourself, what is your attitude toward these systems?

_____

_____

_____

Do you wonder why some policies are in place?

Do you believe in the systems your school has in place?

I want you to take a moment and really think about where you stand on your schools policies.

As an educator you need to, *"consider first, believe in, carry out and be loyal to the established objectives of your institution."* As so beautifully stated by the Cosmetology Educators of America Code of Ethics.

Let me repeat. If you cannot *consider first, believe in, carry out, and be loyal to your institution* you need to find a different career path, whether it is within another school or company.

Listen carefully. By choosing to educate where you are it is your responsibility to abide, cheerfully, to your institution's policies, systems and agreements.

Now, am I saying not to question why policies are in place? Absolutely not. Read your handbooks, yours and your students. Ask questions so that you understand why the policy is in place. Refine them. Is there something that doesn't work? Take the opportunity to reevaluate and make sure your systems are working. You don't have to personally agree with every policy, but you do have to commit to following them faithfully.

Question. What would have happened if, while learning to drive a car, the driving instructor said it didn't matter whether you drove on the left or right side of the road? That just because there was a stop sign didn't mean you had to completely stop, or there was no speed limit or passing lanes on the freeway. I know I wouldn't be a confident driver. I would be scared that I or someone else would be hurt. Driving systems don't change. That's why we can get in you cars every day and travel the world with confidence.

Think of policies, systems and agreements as a safety net. They are there to catch you, not to trap you. Policies, systems and agreements allow you to become everything you aspire to be.

These are some honest responses I've heard from educators when discussing the matter of enforcing policies. "I'm an educator, not a babysitter." Or "I'm paid to teach, not be a hall monitor." These are normal thoughts, so don't feel bad if you've had them too.

But guess what? By enforcing your establishment's policies you're teaching your students a valuable lesson. You're teaching them how to be salon owners, industry educators, great leaders and great employees.

EDUCATORS:

This is the scariest part of becoming a leader and educator. This sets you apart from your peers, and students. If you are not ready for this step, that is okay. There is no judgment here. But there is also no place for you at your establishment at this time. This sounds harsh, and it may be a little tough love, but you cannot run or be part a successful establishment if you are not firm in this area.

If you're ready to be a great leader here's your first challenge: Find out your policies and study them. A true leader doesn't need someone to hand them the policies. They will go to their state licensing website and discover their local regulations. They will study the student handbook, and their own handbook. They will bring to the table discrepancies and always aim to maintain consistency within their environment.

OWNERS/DIRECTORS:

You may have the best team of educators in the world. And I believe you do. But if you have a staff member who will not enforce your policies there is no place at your establishment for them.

Do you know your own policies? Did you write them ten years ago and haven't reviewed them since your last accreditation visit? Know your policies! Review and revise them if necessary.

Quiz your staff and yourself on them regularly and make it a part of your culture.

EDUCATORS, OWNERS AND DIRECTORS:

Are you ready for the paragraph that will change everything?

The beauty of having agreements is that we can manage them perfectly! Yes, you can be a perfect manager! Take the student handbook for example. When your student enrolls, they sign a contract stating that they agree (the agreement) to the policies you've put in place. This takes the person out of it. Wrap your head around this: Your responsibility isn't to manage the person. Your responsibility is to manage the agreement. You can love your student. You can think they are wonderful, creative, and talented, the student you wish you could clone every other student into. But if they show up in brown shoes and your policy says black shoes, you need to send them home. Does this change how you feel about them? Heck no, and you should tell them that. It's not personal, it's the agreement the two of you made before enrollment. There is your simple secret to success. Love your staff and students, make sure they know it and they won't take it personally when you enforce your policies.

I would like to share a personal story with you. I was a school director of a cosmetology school when I talked my baby sister into attending. Now when I say baby sister, I mean I was a teenager when she was born, I treated her like my child and if you ask her to this day she'll claim she has two mothers. Our mother, and myself. I was very clear with her up front that she would be treated just like I treat any other student. My sister, bless her sweet heart, hated to come to school on time. Didn't like working on her mannequin, and loved to hide in the break room and text her friends. Now as part of our school policy, each student was given an advisor, or instructor that they would work with one-on-one. My sister's advisor put her on probation for not staying actively engaged. As part of this probation my sister was given a list of things she needed to accomplish over the following week to "catch up" on. At the end of the week she had not done even half of what she had been advised to accomplish. Her advisor came to me distraught, "What should I do," she asked. "Suspend her" I said matter-of-factly, as this was our policy. "But she's your sister?" "Nope, it's 1 o'clock in the afternoon, she's my student." Now to me, this was not a big deal, but it had a lasting impact on the rest of the student body. The students knew I cared for them, but I also meant business.

Did my sister think she was treated unfairly? No, she thanked me because she wasn't called out for special treatment.

My sister was suspended twice over the course of her program and finished with the minimum amount of requirements she could complete in order to graduate. I am super proud of her and she's a complete success in my eyes.

Staff Project: Gather all your policies and systems in one place such as a large 3 ring binder. This may take time as you review and study your policies and systems. Involve the entire staff.

This binder of policies and systems is the most important tool you have for success. All other things will fall around it. Refer to it often for support.

COSMETOLOGY EDUCATORS OF AMERICA CODE OF ETHICS

As a member of the Cosmetology Educators of America, I hereby pledge my commitment to:

Consider first, believe in, carry out and be loyal to the established objectives of my institution.

Be receptive to competent counsel from colleagues and be guided by such counsel without impairing the dignity and responsibility of the position of an educator.

Pursue continuing knowledge of my career field and maintain practical and current methods of teaching.

Cooperate with professional organizations and individual engaged in activities that enhance the development of cosmetology education.

Be constantly aware of my work methods, self-improvement, and career development opportunities.

Maintain efficiency and consistency in the performance of the administrative tasks of teaching.

Subscribe to and work for honesty and truth in fulfilling the requirements of my position.

Supervise and instruct without prejudice and avoid unethical practices at all times.

Maintain a continuing, realistic analysis and appraisal of the needs of my students.

Counsel and assist fellow instructors in the performance of their duties.

Exhibit a positive, winning attitude and encourage the same in others.

Give a full measure of service in all my endeavors as an educator.

Strive to achieve the highest standards of excellence at all times.

Respect my students, clients, co-workers and fellow educators.

Project a professional image and good grooming at all times.

Create a safe climate and positive learning environment.

Avoid criticism of others and never gossip.

Keep confidentiality where appropriate.

Follow the Golden Rule and be gentle.

Always be punctual and prepared.

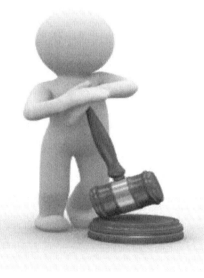

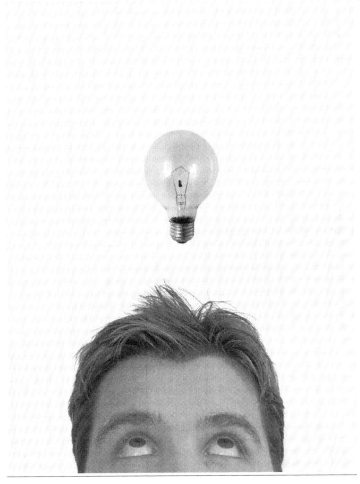

LEADERSHIP JOURNAL

LEADERSHIP JOURNAL

_____

_____

_____

_____

_____

_____

_____

_____

_____

_____

_____

_____

_____

_____

_____

_____

_____

_____

_____

_____

_____

_____

C

CREATE YOUR UNIQUE CULTURE

By believing passionately in something that still does not exist, we create it. The nonexistent is whatever we have not sufficiently desired.

Franz Kafka

How do you differentiate yourself as an establishment from all the other schools out there? Is it a name? Is it a brand? Is it a tradition or ritual?

This is something each school must discover for itself. This will be essential to marketing yourself and ensuring a high student enrollment.

As an educator, what appealed to you about your school? Share this with your owner. Ask your currently enrolled students why they chose you. Brainstorm who you are, or who you'd like to be.

This is another great staff activity, but educators, don't wait for your director or owner to initiate an action of bettering your school. You're a leader now, take it upon yourself to quiz the students or your community. Find out what you're known for and take it back to your school. As a leader it is up to you to stand up and take initiative in bettering yourself and your school. After all, your schools reputation is also your reputation.

Brainstorm the following questions. Keep in mind, not all of these are a must in order for your school to be successful. These questions are just a jumping point to get your mind working. You may have ideas that are different or better than these, you should jot them down and incorporate them!

Does your school have a mission statement or code of ethics?

_____

_____

_____

What curriculum do you use?

_____

_____

_____

Do you develop any of your own curriculum?

_____

_____

_____

Do you partner with industry leaders for hair color, skin care or nails?

_____

_____

_____

Do you bring in outside educators as part of your standard curriculum?

_____

_____

_____

How often do you bring in guest educators?

_____

_____

_____

Do you take your students out on field trips?

_____

_____

_____

Do you have special benchmark projects your students work on? Or a large graduation project?

_____

_____

_____

Do you hold graduation ceremonies?

_____

_____

_____

Do you have any traditions on new start days, such as pancake breakfasts?

_____

_____

_____

Do you participate in any fundraising efforts or local charities?

_____

_____

_____

Do you donate time or services to local organizations?

_____

_____

_____

Do you host runway shows or other events to bring friends and families in?

_____

_____

_____

Does your school keep up with social media marketing such as Facebook or Pinterest?

_____

_____

_____

What are some things you've heard about your surrounding schools, good or bad?

_____

_____

_____

What would you like your graduates to say about you?

_____

_____

_____

What would you like your community to say about you?

_____

_____

_____

This list should give you a start to think about the type of culture you want to create. You may be doing quite a few of these, or none at all. The key to creating your culture, just like your systems, is that they need consistency. Decide carefully what you'd like to incorporate into your culture and then commit to incorporating it.

Use your unique culture as a marketing tool and make sure you tell future students about everything you have to offer.

For some school owners and directors, keeping up with these things are overwhelming in addition to the daily duties of running a school The great news is you now have not only a great staff of educators, but they are also wonderful leaders. Give them the opportunity to step up and take charge of one or two projects.

EDUCATORS:

Don't wait to be asked. What can you offer to your school? This is an amazing way to differentiate yourself.

Staff project:

Set up a yearly calendar with your start dates on it. Try to schedule guest educators a minimum of six months out at a time. Choose some great organizations to celebrate and fundraise for. Think October, breast cancer awareness, November, food drive etc...

Place a large monthly calendar at the beginning of each month where staff and students can see it. This gives students events to look forward to.

OWNERS/ DIRECTORS:

Believe it or not, your educators want to step up. Believe in them. Let go and see what they can do. You'll be surprised and how quickly they take up a leadership role when you allow them to.

Do you have written and outlined job descriptions for each of your employees? If not, involve them in that process. Have each educator write down everything they do on a daily basis for one week. Then have them share what they feel they accomplish that is above and beyond. Lastly, what would they like to do if given the opportunity? Take this feedback and revise your job descriptions.

Do you give your educators titles such as community leader or creative director? These simple titles will give your staff the confidence and boost they need to propel the school. Your community leader could be in charge of completing two fundraising events per year, with your direction and approval. Your creative director could lead your schools runway or fashion show events.

They key to making these educator roles effective is the educators desire. Offer these or other opportunities to only those who want it and can accomplish it in addition to their current educator duties.

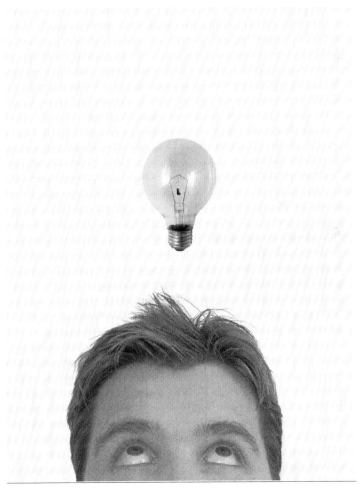

LEADERSHIP JOURNAL

LEADERSHIP JOURNAL

_____

_____

_____

_____

_____

_____

_____

_____

_____

_____

_____

_____

_____

_____

_____

_____

_____

_____

_____

_____

_____

_____

_____

_____

_____

DON'T SWEAT THE SMALL STUFF- IT'S NOT ALL SMALL STUFF.

Little minds have little worries, big minds have no time for worries.

Ralph Waldo Emerson

Leadership Tip: Leaders aren't perfect.

Your school is never going to be perfect. Your students are never going to be perfect. You are never going to be perfect.

You want to hear the number one concern I hear from students? "There's no consistency in my school!"

See? That one statement just made your pulse race and sent blood rising to your brain. Am I right?

You want to scream through the pages right now. "We are consistent!!! Those students wouldn't know consistency if it hit them in the face. We work so hard on consistency and they don't appreciate anything we do. I give up!"

Think about this next statement for a moment… You may be consistent in enforcing your policies, but are you consistent in *THE WAY* you enforce your policies? Aha! Simply put, when it comes to consistency, our students not only judge us on our follow through. But *HOW THEY FELT* when we followed through. Aren't we an emotional bunch?

You're going to hear me say this over and over again. It's the beauty of having all those agreements we've been talking about, and why they are so important. As hard as it is for us to not take our students words and actions personally, you must not let that interfere with your leadership. Remember, your job is to manage the agreements, and you need to be kind with your students while doing it. Great leaders don't show their frustration, anger or sadness while managing or leading their group (although they have the same feelings the rest of us do). Start practicing your poker face. When you take your emotions out of it you'll notice the rants of inconsistencies start to cease.

This can be extremely difficult. So how do we do this?

Let's start by how we don't do this. We are more easily affected by negative emotions than we are positive ones. Try not to get wrapped up in the little day-to-day dramas that surround your students. Don't listen in on any negative gossip or opinions unless you're directly responsible for handling it. Don't add your opinion on personal matters. Keep yourself emotionally distant from your student's personal lives. Note: Emotionally distant from your student's personal lives is vastly different than not being wholeheartedly invested in their professional success.

Take a break if you need to. Go into your broom closet, shut the door and hit your head against the wall a few times if you have to. Breathe. It's okay.

Step back and look at the big picture. Your primary focus is to give them a great education. Teach them responsibility and business skills. Ensure they graduate, test out, and are placed in a salon or industry related field. When you get caught up in an emotional meltdown, remember this sentence. It will help you refocus.

Pick your battles. Go back to your policies, manage your agreements (every single time), follow your systems, and let the rest go.

There are going to be days when a student may do something that irritates the hell out of you. Maybe it was bad, maybe it wasn't really a big deal. Maybe no one else would even notice the behavior and that student just happened to rub you the wrong way. How do you respond to this student? Most of us (because we're human) will try to enforce a disciplinary action towards that student for a policy that doesn't' exist. In other words, you want to do something but don't have a policy or system in place to back you up. You need to let it go.

If it is something that you feel strongly needs to be placed in your policies, take it back to your team. But without a policy in place you have no leg to stand on. I repeat. Let it go.

By enforcing policies and only policies with kindness and fairness it builds trust between the school, the staff, and the students. This trust is what allows the magic of learning to happen and you'll be able to focus on giving your students the best education you have to offer.

There are days when you're going to hurt. Not the physical standing on your feet kind of hurt (although there's plenty of those too). But the emotional, heart wrenching, knot in your throat kind of hurt.

There is going to be days you question why you wanted to become an educator. Why you don't feel like you're making a difference. Why no one listens to you, or respects you, or heck, even likes you.

Why am I telling you this? I have no magic formula to ensure this never happens. But I'm sharing this so that you know that we all have these days and you're not alone.

You are making a difference.

You are changing lives.

And you know what else? Tomorrow will come, you'll wake up with dry eyes and ready to do it again.

So in case you don't hear it enough, which you won't, thank you! Thank you for making our profession the greatest one in the world! There are no cosmetologists, estheticians, nail techs, barbers, schools, salons, or educators without you. Think about that!

LEADERSHIP JOURNAL

LEADERSHIP JOURNAL

_____

_____

_____

_____

_____

_____

_____

_____

_____

_____

_____

_____

_____

_____

_____

_____

_____

_____

_____

_____

_____

_____

_____

_____

_____

ELEVATE YOURSELF.

I know of no more encouraging fact than the unquestionable ability of man to elevate his life by conscious endeavor.

Henry David Thoreau

By elevating yourself, I mean that you are not on the same level as your students. If you were to picture an organizational chart in your head, this is what it might look like. You see the Owner or Director above you and the students below you and yourself right smack in the middle. You may feel like you're the liaison between the two and if you're to be completely honest, you might feel closer to the student side than the management side. Am I right? Let me paint a picture for you just so we're clear.

Cosmetology school flow chart from an educator's perspective:

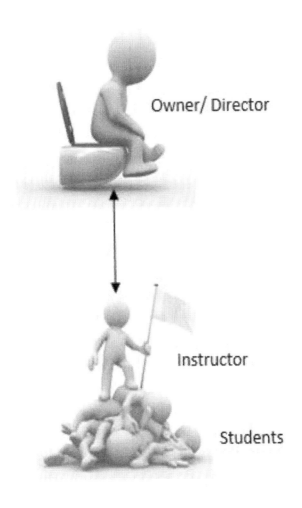

Owner/ Director

Instructor

Students

Now let me paint you a different picture.

Cosmetology school flow chart from an owner/director perspective:

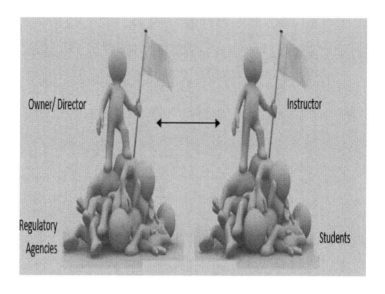

Why are these so different? But more importantly, whose perspective needs to change?

These pictures are humorous, but they also paint a real picture. A picture that damages a lot of schools. It is a great divide of minds that can wreak havoc in schools.

Let me clear up the thought process of both sides, because I've been on both sides. Let's start with the instructor's perspective. From where you sit, you are in the trenches. You are dealing with the policies that the directors are telling you to manage. Here is some of the thoughts that run through your head on a daily basis.

"I don't see **them** having to tell students to put away their cell phones or get working on their mannequins all day long."

"Must be nice to be able to leave for lunch when you want to."

"I wish **I** could sit behind a computer, or in meetings all day."

"The tuition is going up again? I wonder where all the money is going, it certainly isn't coming to me."

"Grrr…"

Now, some of you may not ever entertain thoughts like these, and I'm certainly not trying to clump all educators together, nor am I saying that these are bad thoughts (Alright, I am. But we've all thought them.). I'm simply speaking for the majority of instructors I've worked with.

Only you can answer how you feel within your own organization.

Here are some thoughts from an owner or director's perspective.

"*Bleeping* regulatory agencies are changing things again?!?!"

"It's so nice to have a team I can trust, so I can get these things done"

"I hope my instructors know how much I appreciate them."

"It's going to take the next ten years to get these IPEDS done!"

"Grrr..."

I promise you, contrary to some people's beliefs, owners never have thoughts like this:

"I'm off to have a seven-course lunch while my minions work to collect me more money. Bwahahahaha…"

"If I can hold off giving pay raises for 5 more years I'll be able to afford that private island I've always dreamed of. Bwahahahaha…."

Here is the truth from both sides. Everyone is over-worked and under-appreciated at times.

We don't readily see the work or commitment everyone puts into his or her day.

We all have a darn hard job.

So what can we do to see eye to eye? Are you ready for the answer?

EDUCATORS:

You are a leader. You were hired to do a job (educate and manage agreements). You do your job well, and I hope your owner or director can appreciate you in whatever way helps to validate you.

You are an equal, a partner with your school. Although you are an advocate for your students, you are hired to **consider first, believe in, carry out and be loyal to the established objectives of your institution.**

The hardest part of being a leader is to realize you might have been on the wrong side of the fence for a majority of your teaching career. But hurry up, it's not too late to open the gate and walk on through.

SCHOOL DIRECTORS/OWNERS:

I know you feel like you validate your staff constantly by telling them they are amazing. Why isn't that working? There is a mistrust that runs rampant between owners and instructors. Whether you intend it or not? So what are you doing wrong? Nothing. What can you do better?

COMMUNICATE. This is the number cause of mistrust between you and your educators. You need to be in constant communication. Build a relationship of trust with them. They need to feel they can talk with you openly and honestly. How do you do this? There are a few different methods you can begin with. The first is as much as you tell your staff to be consistent with policies and agreements. You must do the same. If you say you're going to meet with your staff once a week then you must do it. If you say you're going to evaluate your staff on a particular day, or have annual reviews by a certain day. Do it. We sometimes unintentionally blow off our staff if something that seems more important comes up, we figure we'll have time later. You have no staff if you have no trust.

The second piece of advice I'd like to share is to make yourself approachable. Are you so overwhelmed that you snap when a question or concern is brought up? Do you get frustrated when your staff involves you with "petty" student issues instead of handling it themselves? Do you support your instructors if they've made a mistake?

If you take the time to help your staff work through concerns they have with patience and kindness, your staff will feel safe. They will come to you less often with concerns because they will feel confident they're doing things right. They will know with certainty that it's okay to make mistakes and that you will be there to coach them and support them.

EDUCATORS:

One more thing…. Take the above piece of advice and apply it to your students.

The correct perspective:

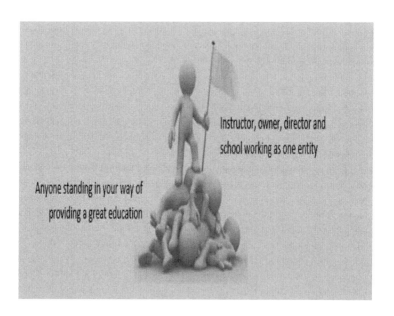

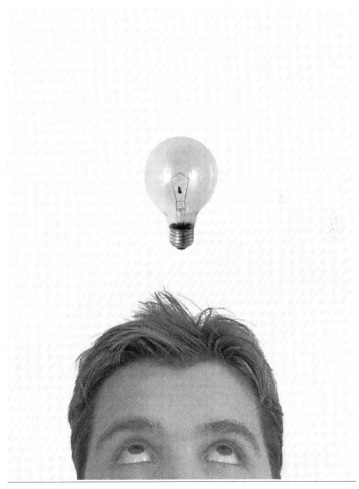

LEADERSHIP JOURNAL

LEADERSHIP JOURNAL

_____

_____

_____

_____

_____

_____

_____

_____

_____

_____

_____

_____

_____

_____

_____

_____

_____

_____

_____

_____

_____

_____

_____

_____

_____

_____

FOLLOW THE LEADER. OH WAIT- THAT'S YOU!

If your actions inspire others to dream more, learn more, do more and become more, you are a leader.

John Quincy Adams

Remember growing up and running into one of your teacher's at the grocery store or restaurant. Do you remember thinking, "That's weird. I didn't know they ate". When you think more about it, we never expected our teachers to actually be a real person, with a life and a family. We thought they only existed between the hours of 7:30 a.m. to 3:30 p.m., and then "poof", they disappeared until tomorrow.

You should only exist for your students 8 hours a day.

Trust me, your students all want to be your friend. They will invite you to their showers, jewelry parties, New Year's Parties, and any other occasion they can find to hang out with you. By being an educator you automatically have a cool factor that your students want to be around.

But guess what? Your students have plenty of people around them to be friends with. They don't need another friend. They need someone to look up to. Someone that can mentor them and be a good role-model. Your career path not only consists of teaching them how to palm their shears, but also how to respect themselves, their peers and their future employers. While they are in school you fill the "boss" role. This an excellent learning opportunity for them to cultivate a professional working relationship. Remember although we get students from all walks of life, we deal with a lot of student's fresh out of high school, without a lot of real life, grown up, professional relationships. School should be a safe place for them to develop these types of relationships. They will learn that everyone does not have to be a personal friend in order to develop deep and respectful connections.

There is a line that must be clearly defined. And if you want to save yourself a lot of trouble you will stay on your side of the no-friend zone.

Most schools already have this policy in place. If yours doesn't, put it in place right now. Then when they ask you to join in their after school activities, you can simply say, "That sounds like fun, but It's against school policy for me to meet you outside of school." Again, it comes back to managing an agreement. You didn't have to say, "I don't want to be your friend." Or "Why would I want to go to your shower?"

By following the no-friend policy it helps us to manage our agreements with our students. You can also leave any personal knowledge you might gain, or unprofessional emotional connections out of your decision making.

Some of you might find drawing the line hard. You may crave the friendship and camaraderie your students give to you. Others feel like the student's will behave better for them if you have a personal relationship.

Again, it goes back to the career you've chosen. If you want to make personal friendships, you might find working in a salon a better fit for you.

No-friend zone advice: Some schools have their student's call their instructors Mr. or Mrs. <name>. By addressing your instructors in a professional manner such as this it enforces a professional relationship.

The good news is, even if you have been feeling a little too friendly with your students, it's never too late to make a commitment to yourself to reexamine your role in their life, you can start over right now and become the leader they need.

One more piece of leadership advice on talking to our student's about policies: As a society we love to break rules. Why? Because we don't like rules.

Consider the word "rule" as taboo as saying pluck, dye, and bleach or "I just use Suave".

Our students will respect the idea that we have policies to adhere to much more than the idea of having "rules" to follow.

LEADERSHIP JOURNAL

LEADERSHIP JOURNAL

_____

_____

_____

_____

_____

_____

_____

_____

_____

_____

_____

_____

_____

_____

_____

_____

_____

_____

_____

_____

_____

_____

_____

_____

G

GATHER FOR YOUR TRIBE.

We spent an enormous amount of time as hominids and as primates living as hunter-gatherers. That is the natural way for us to live, and we're suddenly living in this profoundly unnatural way, and we're still in the process of adapting to it and working out how to live with it.

Spencer Wells

As an educator, you most likely have been given a curriculum outline and asked to follow it in your classes. This is great, and the way a good system works.

You may take for granted the day-to-day decisions that have been made on behalf of your institution, such as:

Why did we decide to use this color line or skin care line?

Why do we carry the books we carry in our library?

Why do teach a pedicure the way we teach it.

We just go with the flow, never questioning why we do what we do. We become a good employee, and educator, but this manual is about developing leaders.

Again I'm going to ask you to change your perspective. As an educator, you are the leader of your own tribe of students. You are the hunter and the gatherer. It is your duty to provide for your students. No, we are not talking about physical food, we are talking about brain food.

Discover the why behind why you do what you do, and why you use what you use. Make it a mission to understand why you educate the way you do. What the decision making process is behind why you choose one product line over another. Do they offer perks? Complimentary education?

When we understand and feel confident about all aspects of what we do and why we do it, things make more sense to us. After all, you've heard the old saying. You don't know what you don't know.

What are you personally doing to gather knowledge to take back to your tribe? If your waiting for your school owner to send you to a class, that's great. But it's also like the hunter waiting for the buffalo to come to him. It could happen, but it's going to take a lot longer than if you took the initiative to make things happen yourself. What can YOU do?

Can you commit to attending hair shows?

Could you attend a yearly CEA convention?

Is there a new skill you'd like to learn such as hair or lash extensions, chemical peels, speed waxing, or another cosmetology related skill?

Can you email product companies you're already using and ask if they are developing any new products? Do they have any online resources or complimentary downloads you can pass on to your students?

Can you email companies you're not currently using and ask them to send you information? Take your new information and turn it into a student activity. Compare and contrast them. Divide into groups and ask each group to present a 15 minute mini class.

Ask guest educators how they got their start and why they chose to represent their respected companies. Perhaps you could schedule 3 or 4 on the same day and have students interview them.

Go visit salons and speak with the owners, find out what they're looking for in their new hires. Have they hired any of your graduates? Were they happy with their decision? Why or why not? Do they have any advice on what they would like your students to know or feel more comfortable in before they are salon ready?

By fulfilling the role of the gatherer you are keeping your students sustained. People are just as happy with a full mind as they are a full belly.

Never become complacent in your career. There is always something new and innovative in the industry. Be an example to your students and show them that they should never be done learning.

What are some ideas of ways you can gather new information for your team?

LEADERSHIP JOURNAL

_____

_____

_____

_____

_____

_____

_____

_____

_____

_____

_____

_____

_____

_____

_____

_____

_____

_____

LEADERSHIP JOURNAL

_____

_____

_____

_____

_____

_____

_____

_____

_____

_____

_____

_____

_____

_____

_____

_____

_____

_____

_____

_____

_____

_____

_____

HIDE AND SEEK IS NOT JUST FOR KIDS.

To succeed, jump as quickly at opportunities as you do at conclusions.

Benjamin Franklin

Opportunities are all around you. Little gems of knowledge and friendships and experiences.

Where are they? They are normally right in front of you, hidden in plain sight. Opportunities can be found easily if you open yourself up to the possibility of finding them.

You normally wouldn't go looking for your brother in the kitchen cabinet, but when it comes to hide and seek you do. You start looking in places you didn't know existed.

Opportunities work the same way. Where are you looking? If you're living your everyday life looking in the same places you've always looked there's a chance an opportunity may eventually come knocking. But the chances of this are the same as your single friend who really wants a relationship but won't leave her house. Has her future husband come knocking yet? Probably not.

The easiest way to look for opportunities is through people. Start building connections and networking. You'll find we all have the same dreams and desires and it's very easy to connect with others in our industry. LinkedIn is a great place to find opportunities and friendships. Get yourself noticed by participating in chats and discussions. There are also a lot of professional groups you can join on Facebook.

A lot of industry greats got their starts through social media.

Do you or your school have a YouTube channel? That's an excellent place to begin to get noticed.

What about a personal blog that you can add to your business card. And speaking of business cards, are you handing them out?

Vendors at shows love if we introduce ourselves as instructors or educators. You'll normally walk away with twice as much information and samples as anyone else. Take their business cards and email them after the show. Ask questions and thank them for taking the time to speak with you.

It's very easy to start forming a vast network of support around you. This becomes crucial as a leader, you will get to know many people, who will introduce you to other people, who will introduce you to other people. After this you can sit in your house like your single friend and opportunities will literally come knocking at your door.

We've talked about how imperative it is to not cultivate "friendships" with your students. As a result of this, being an educator can feel a bit lonely. There are thousands of people in your industry just like you who feel the same way. By putting yourself out there you will develop more sincere, long-lasting friendships than you've ever dreamed of. This can be extremely rewarding. And when you have a bad day, and you can't talk to your "student friend" about it, think how grateful you'll feel for all the genuine support you've built.

Activity: Google yourself. What images come up? Hopefully none from your bachelorette party. Is there any information about you positive or negative?

Professionals seeking out other professionals for opportunities will generally google that person for information. Remember you are a professional. Be cautious what you post in your personal media. These words and images can come back to haunt you.

What if there is nothing? Well that's okay, but I have a trick for you (of course I do).

Besides having a LinkedIn account, Blog, or professional Facebook page (which I hope you have all three), offer to write testimonials for your product manufacturers. If they post your testimonial on their website it will generate your name in a search.

Marketing yourself professionally through social media is the number one way to get yourself out there!

One last thing hide and seekers: You and your other educators should work hard to build yourself as one strong united team. You will be each other's biggest support system. Your team is not your competition. There is no reward for favorite instructor, no reward for least favorite instructor. There is no reward for suck-ups and no reward for lazy instructor. You need to all be on the same bus, not throwing each other under it. If you're having disagreements or differences within your organization you need to learn how to communicate clearly, hold each other accountable and fix it. Make an agreement this very second that you will not speak about each other behind backs. If you need to clarify something you will go directly to that educator, and only that educator. Period. Agreed?

And speaking of this very subject let's move on to the next chapter.

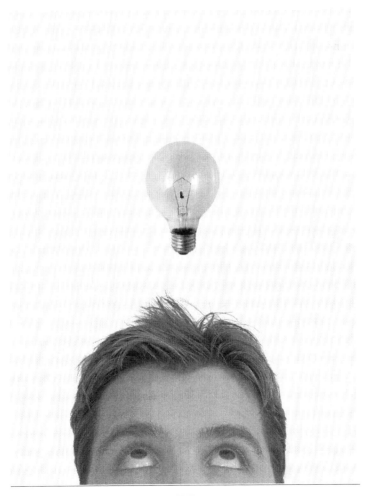

LEADERSHIP JOURNAL

LEADERSHIP JOURNAL

_____
_____
_____
_____
_____
_____
_____
_____
_____
_____
_____
_____
_____
_____
_____
_____
_____
_____
_____
_____
_____
_____
_____
_____
_____

I

INTEGRITY IS THE MOST VALUABLE FORM OF CURRENCY.

Real integrity is doing the right thing, knowing that nobody's going to know whether you did it or not.

Oprah Winfrey

Integrity

1. The quality of being honest and having strong moral principles; moral uprightness

2. The state of being whole and undivided.

Hmm. The quality of being honest and having strong moral principles. Let's delve a little deeper.

Principles

1. the principles of right and wrong that are accepted by an individual or a social group;

This is the definition of the word integrity. What are the principles of right and wrong in your personal definition of integrity? Note: this is personal and there are no wrong answers.

_____

_____

_____

_____

_____

Look at your answers. Do you embody your definition of integrity? Why or why not?

_____

_____

_____

_____

_____

Think of five people you know, admire, and respect.

_____

_____

_____

_____

_____

What do you admire and respect about them?

_____

_____

_____

_____

_____

How do they make you feel?

_____

_____

_____

_____

_____

How do they make others feel?

_____

_____

_____

_____

_____

What traits do they have in common?

_____

_____

_____

_____

_____

Do these people have integrity according to your definition?

_____

_____

_____

_____

_____

Would you offer them the gift of time, knowledge, help or assistance if they needed it? What would you ask for in return?

_____

_____

_____

_____

_____

Chances are you said yes, you would offer them all of the above if they asked for it and you would not ask anything in return.

So if we are willing to offer something to these five people you've listed without an exchange or return, why would we do it? Love? Respect? Admiration?

Yes.

But we would also do these things for the feelings we receive when we give something of value (yes, your time, knowledge, help and assistance are all valuable) for nothing. We need these feelings as much as we need sunshine, and fresh air and clean water. These feelings make us feel alive, worthy, powerful and happy.

So why aren't we walking around giving ourselves to everyone without wanting anything in return?

Simply stated, we don't like to give things to people we don't feel have integrity. People that we don't love, respect or admire. People without integrity wouldn't appreciate those gifts or see value in them, therefor we don't get the same feeling of joy as when we give to those we respect and care about.

Have you ever heard the saying, "You get what you give."?
If you can form the same traits as those you've listed above do you believe people would give those same gifts freely to you?

Open yourself up to continually elevating your integrity. Live in a way that brings you peace, joy and happiness. You will find that you will attract the same type of people as yourself. You will find you have a lot to offer in the way of support, friendship, and the sharing of knowledge and in return the same will be given to you. These moments of sharing and support become as strong and solid as rungs on a ladder. Each opportunity allows you to climb one step higher to your dream of leadership.

Believe this my friends, nothing on this earth will ever get you further or be more valuable than your integrity. Cultivate it, practice it, live it and breathe it.

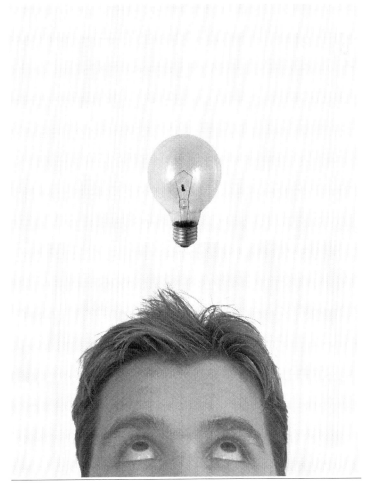

LEADERSHIP JOURNAL

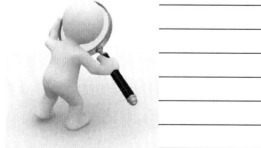

LEADERSHIP JOURNAL

_____

_____

_____

_____

_____

_____

_____

_____

_____

_____

_____

_____

_____

_____

_____

_____

_____

_____

_____

_____

_____

_____

_____

_____

J

JUGGLING IS FOR CLOWNS.

"Don't say you don't have enough time. You have exactly the same number of hours per day that were given to Helen Keller, Pasteur, Michelangelo, Mother Teresa, Leonardo da Vinci, Thomas Jefferson, and Albert Einstein."

H. Jackson Brown, Jr.

By this point in our journey, I hope you're feeling a bit inspired and more confident in yourself and your abilities. It's also about the time that reality loves to come in and squash us.

Do you feel as if you're taking one step forward and two steps back? You may also feel that as much as you want these newly discovered leadership skills, there is always something or someone standing in your way.

Do you feel like you're stuck in a revolving door with no way out? Do you feel like you come to work, clock in, step on the proverbial hamster wheel and stay there until it's time to clock out?

There has to be progress in order to produce momentum. And we need momentum to keep propelling us forward.

There are some days that it takes everything in us to just put a smile on our face, let alone work on our leadership progression.

Overwhelmed is a word that can be used to describe us on an everyday basis. I cannot reiterate enough how tough of a career path you've chosen. You are responsible to calculate complicated color formulas in ounces, help wrap a yellow and blue rod perm, answer questions on why your students are not allowed to have their cell phones out on the student salon and sooth a crying two year old getting his hair cut… all at the same time. It's a wonder that we have the ability to get out of bed in the morning.

So how do we juggle it all?

We don't. Yes, there are times when you feel like you have ten balls in the air, let them fall.

In reality, we aren't clowns, contrary to our student's beliefs.

Start bowling instead.

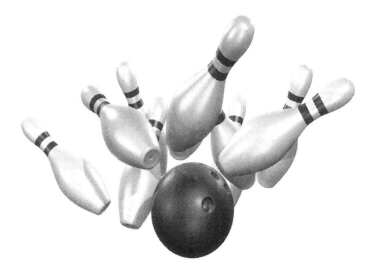

See all those pins (things to do) down the lane? Those are your day-to day scenarios that we all have to deal with. Now get your nice eight-pound ball and knock them down with one strike.

How do we do this?

Line up what you need to accomplish in the morning with the help of a "to do" list. Line them up in the order you're most likely to strike them (order of importance) and give it your best shot.

Don't go into your day blindly, with no plan as to what you wish to accomplish. Everyday should have a plan. Refer to your job description if need be.

Organize your duties into a list of what needs to get done on a daily, weekly, or monthly basis.

Could you incorporate a rotation of coverage that would allow all your educators to have 30 minutes a day to plan lessons, complete extra responsibilities, answer emails, contact suppliers, journal, work on personal development, or just decompress?

An important key to success as a leader and educator is focus and time management.

Keep your mind focused on your goals and don't lose sight of them. It's a lot easier to line up your pins (goals) and focus on knocking as many of them down as you can,

than it is to throw them up in the air and hope you catch
them.

And although it seems that the time we have does not
belong to us, this is a great opportunity to come together
as a team and work together to help each other
accomplish our goals.

When your staff respect and value each other enough to
make time for one another, everyone wins.

Remember the previous chapter on integrity? Offer to
cover for your team to help them accomplish their goals
and they will offer to cover for you.

You'll be amazed at how much more you get
accomplished and how much less stress you feel when
you have a daily plan.

Daily Duties:

_____

_____

_____

_____

_____

_____

_____

_____

_____

_____

_____

_____

_____

_____

_____

_____

_____

_____

_____

_____

_____

Weekly Duties:

_____

_____

_____

_____

_____

_____

_____

_____

Monthly Duties:

_____

_____

_____

_____

_____

_____

_____

_____

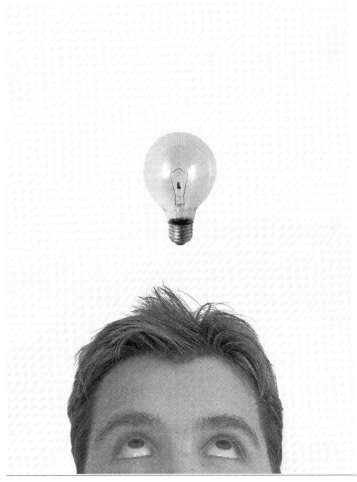

LEADERSHIP JOURNAL

LEADERSHIP JOURNAL

_____

_____

_____

_____

_____

_____

_____

_____

_____

_____

_____

_____

_____

_____

_____

_____

_____

_____

_____

_____

_____

_____

KINDNESS IN EVERYTHING.

Kindness is the language which the deaf can hear and the blind can see.

Mark Twain

As simplistic as this idea sounds. Kindness does not come easy to everyone.

As an educator, you've probably heard some of the backgrounds your students come from. The hardships they've faced. The trials they've overcome.

You might have also weathered some pretty rough storms in your own life.

Here is a story Stephen Covey shared in his book, The Seven Habits of Highly Effective People.

"I remember a mini-Paradigm Shift I experienced one Sunday morning on a subway in New York. People were sitting quietly -- some reading newspapers, some lost in thought, some resting with their eyes closed. It was a calm, peaceful scene. Then suddenly, a man and his children entered the subway car. The children were so loud and rambunctious that instantly the whole climate changed.

"The man sat down next to me and closed his eyes, apparently oblivious to the situation. The children were yelling back and forth, throwing things, even grabbing people's papers. It was very disturbing. And yet, the man sitting next to me did nothing.

"It was difficult not to feel irritated. I could not believe that he could be so insensitive to let his children run wild like that and do nothing about it, taking no responsibility at all. It was easy to see that everyone else on the subway felt irritated, too. So finally, with what I felt was unusual patience and restraint, I turned to him and said, "Sir, your children are really disturbing a lot of people. I wonder if you couldn't control them a little more."

"The man lifted his gaze as if to come to a consciousness of the situation for the first time and said softly, 'Oh, you're right. I guess I should do something about it. We just came from the hospital where their mother died about an hour ago. I don't know what to think, and I guess they don't know how to handle it either.'

"Can you imagine what I felt at that moment? My paradigm shifted. Suddenly I saw things differently, I felt differently, I behaved differently. My irritation vanished. I didn't have to worry about controlling my attitude or my behavior; my heart was filled with the man's pain. Feelings of sympathy and compassion flowed freely. "Your wife just died? Oh, I'm so sorry. Can you tell me about it? What can I do to help?" Everything changed in an instant."

Have you ever found yourself in a similar situation?

This powerful change of attitude and behavior was the result of his discovery of information that he hadn't known before. Once he understood the situation, his attitude became caring and his behavior became helpful.

Sadly for us, we won't always have the gift of discovering information. Most times, we won't know why people will behave the way that they do, nor is it our job to judge why people behave the way that they do.

The truth is, we don't know what trials our students are enduring in or out of school.

We make a lot of assumptions. This is a good student, this is a bad student. What do we do when a "good" student needs disciplinary action? Do you give them a break? Perhaps turn a blind eye or sweep it under the rug? I'm not going to answer this question because you already know what the answer should be.

What about a "bad" student, do you huff and puff and glare and think to yourself, "Why do they always make things so difficult for everyone?"

What if we knew the inner motives and feelings of our students, most people aren't "bad" on purpose. What if only saw our student's positive personality traits. Everyone has "good" in them. Do you think we would feel more compassionate? Do you think it would help us to manage agreements with love instead of accusations?

When leading your students you must adapt an attitude of kindness. This means that although you might not agree with their behavior and must manage the agreement that has been made between you. Your feelings of respect and love for them don't change. Their behavior bears no reflection in the way you feel about them as a person. You acknowledge that everyone has valuable characteristics and deserves to be treated fairly and kindly.

Consider this:

When "good" students discover they can get away with things and aren't disciplined for it they become "bad" students.

When "bad" students discover that you treat them just as kindly and fairly as everyone else they become "good" students."

By being consistent with all of your students, no matter what, they all become "good" students.

People are like prisms. Everyone contains within them beautiful rainbows of ideas and concepts and wisdom and knowledge just waiting to for the right person to shine a little light on them. There is nothing more beautiful than watching the colors of enlightenment burst out of a person who has been in the shadows for too long.

Practicing kindness makes your inner light shine brighter? Can you feel it? Take your light and shine it on others. Especially those who might have grown dim, withdrawn, secluded or lonely?

How do you do this? Exactly as you have been. Show people how wonderful they are by acknowledging them in positive ways every chance that you get. Tell them how talented and wonderful they are. Show them a new technique and cheer them on as they master it.

Here are a few ways that can help you develop an attitude of kindness within your school:

Smile. At everyone, every day.

Reach out to at least one student every day and try to connect with them on a personal level. Even saying hello can mean the world to a student that's having a bad day.

For every piece of constructive criticism you dish out to your students, tell them something they're doing right.

Notice friendly or helpful behavior among your students or staff and acknowledge it, publicly if possible. Being recognized for our good behavior only makes us want to do it more.

Never discipline a student or acknowledge bad behavior publicly. Pull them aside privately. This shows that you respect them and care for their feelings.

Being kind does not mean that we can't teach our student's. You still need to be as firm in your teaching as you are in managing your agreements. This means correcting student's practical abilities and theory skills when they need it.

Being kind does not mean "sugar coating" everything. Our students crave feedback. We need to correct them and challenge them in order for them to grow and push themselves. You will find that your students will seek you out for feedback if you can do it honestly and kindly.

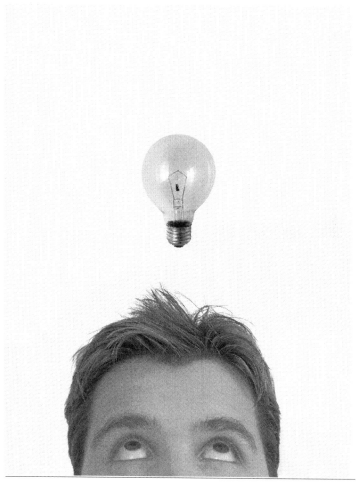

LEADERSHIP JOURNAL

LEADERSHIP JOURNAL

_____

_____

_____

_____

_____

_____

_____

_____

_____

_____

_____

_____

_____

_____

_____

_____

_____

_____

_____

_____

_____

_____

_____

LOVE YOURSELF. A LOT.

I have an everyday religion that works for me. Love yourself first, and everything else falls into line.

Lucille Ball

We are nearly half way through our leadership training. How do you feel?

This is the perfect time to congratulate yourself on all of your hard work. You are probably starting to notice things falling into place. You may be experiencing a little momentum in your career and hopefully a lot of confidence.

You also might be beginning to notice some of your relationships changing and evolving as people are now looking up to you as a leader. Take a moment to reflect on the positive changes that have been happening in your career.

_____

_____

_____

_____

_____

I am proud of you and all the changes you've made. If I could give you any reward for all your hard work I would give you the ability to love yourself. A lot.

Ever notice how much easier it is for us to love other people unconditionally, but we point out our own flaws incessantly.

Just as much as we need to acknowledge others for their positive behavior, you need to acknowledge yourself for just how amazing you are.

How do you appreciate yourself? Everyone loves

themselves and others in different ways. Find what makes you tick and reward yourself with it.

Perhaps you could develop a Sunday night ritual. Invest in an at-home spa experience. Light candles, use bath salts or oils, maybe a new scrub and mask for your face, grab a glass of wine and check out a juicy romance novel from the library. Make sure you have a fluffy white spa robe and towels when you get out. Now that's my idea of an amazing night loving myself.

My guilty pleasure is self-help or motivational books. I love to buy these and read them reverently. After I place them on a special bookshelf. When I re-read these books I'm always taken back to when I purchased them and the reward I've given myself.

Maybe books don't do it for you and that's okay. Buy yourself that pair of shoes or new outfit you've been wanting.

Schedule yourself a monthly massage, facial or pedicure.

Take a weekend and watch an entire television series on Netflix while eating a few pints of Ben & Jerry's.

Take yourself snowboarding or register for an art class

If you take the time to love yourself you will find it much easier to love your career, your family, and your relationships.

List five ways in which you can love yourself, and start implementing them, right now.

_____

_____

_____

_____

_____

LEADERSHIP JOURNAL

LEADERSHIP JOURNAL

M

MAKING MONEY IS THEIR GOAL

Money won't create success, the freedom to make it will.

Nelson Mandela

Although this book is primarily about self-leadership, we still have a school to run and successful students to graduate and employ. Part of this personal journey is to constantly and consistently use the skills you are learning to ensure your students get the very best education you can give them.

Sometimes we forget why our students enrolled in school. If it's not to make money than they need to reevaluate their career path.

It is essential for every school to establish a business course. Your students not only need to learn how to section hair and polish nails, but they need to know how to make money while doing it.

In order for them to build a successful business, it takes above all, leadership skills. Who better than you to share with them how to become a leader? By teaching others how to become leaders, it makes you a better leader.

You can use a lot of the concepts you've been learning in this book and apply it right in your own business course.

Here are a few topics your students should be learning in order to be successful in their career paths.

- Customer service skills. We may take for granted meeting, relating to, and serving clients, but some of our students have never done this before. Do your student's shake their guest's hands? Do they walk beside them to their stations? Do they speak in a clear voice? Do they use eye contact? Do they focus 100% on their guests and not on their neighbors or friends? Begin with the basics of how to connect with people and develop good client/stylist relationships.

- Communication skills. Great consultation skills begin with great communication skills. I suggest incorporating as many communication activities as you can. Google communication activities for lots of great ideas. Practice often.

- Confidence, or the ability to "fake it till you make it". How do we instill confidence? By letting them discover and try, and make mistakes, and see their brilliance. We do our student's no service by giving them busy-work or by not allowing them to try new things. Let them color and perm and cut their mannequins. Let them try formulating client colors on their own. Encourage them to try new techniques or products. Let them get their hands dirty and play. People learn by doing. You've heard it before, but it's true, busy students are happy students and the harder they work the more confidence they gain.

- Retail skills. Do they have professional products to use on clients? Do you bring in educators to teach about these products? In order to be a successful stylist your students must know how to retail products. We all know this, but it's such a hard concept to teach. Does your computer system calculate retail to service percentages? Because school services are priced so reasonably, it is fairly easy for student stylists to meet a goal of 10% retail to service. Perhaps you could print off certificates each month for every student who meets this goal. Have them place them in their portfolios. Explain how this will help them edge out competition when looking for employment.

- Pre-booking. This is another big area lacking in schools and salons alike. But successful stylists know that this is really the number one key to success. Did you know that clients who pre-book normally visit the salon up to 20% more times a year than client's who don't pre-book? Take haircuts for example. If a client pre-books every 4 weeks, they will receive 13 haircuts a year. Let's say that same faithful client doesn't pre-book but calls when he's ready. This averages out to about one haircut every 5 weeks. Now that client is only receiving 10 haircuts a year. Those missed haircuts could add up to $100.00 or more. And that's just one client! Imagine you have 20 clients that don't pre-book. That's a lost income of $2,000 dollars a year. Now we took the example of a haircut which is a lower priced service. You could work out these same scenarios with hair color or other higher priced services. Always show your students the value in what they're missing. Show them what the information could mean to them. Script your students and make it a habit to ask their clients to pre-book.

- Referral programs. Show them techniques that work when asking clients for referrals. Role-play scenarios so it won't feel uncomfortable for them to ask. Place it in a script along with the above information and make it part of their grade.

- Tracking services and setting goals. Have your students take their daily, and weekly services and figure out their pay for the week. Research different salons in your area. The service prices, and how their stylists are paid. Use this information and have them take their weekly services and pay themselves according to the salon's pay scales. Have your student's write themselves fake paychecks. And once a month have your students pay their bills with them. They need to have a realistic idea of how much work it's going to take them to succeed. This will also help them determine where they might like to work and help them set goals to achieve working at their dream job.

These are just a few ideas, I'm sure you have many more that are just as great and valuable. Now put them together with your team and make a plan. Commit to incorporating them into your culture.

Take some time to look at your curriculum as a whole. Are your students confident and busy? What are they learning? Are they consistently producing good work?

Push, push, push your students to do and be better each day. Don't become complacent in your school or teaching methods.

LEADERSHIP JOURNAL

LEADERSHIP JOURNAL

NO IS AN OKAY WORD.

The art of leadership is saying no, not saying yes. It is very easy to say yes.

Tony Blair

Why do we find it so hard to say no?

Look how great your students have been? It's slow on the student salon, and although it's against your policy, don't they deserve to get a spa day on the clock?

No.

See that wasn't so hard, was it?

Alright, it *is* hard. There are times when all is well, everyone has been actively engaged. Your team is getting along better than ever. All the stars have aligned and it seems like you've finally got everything under control.

Feels good, doesn't it?

Guess what happens when we feel good? We let our guards down. We start thinking crazy thoughts such as, "We can let a few things slip every once in a while, we haven't been having any problems. Surely it's not a big deal if we ignore the policy this one time. It's a special day. The student body we have right now wouldn't dream of taking advantage of us."

I know you've been there so I don't even need to tell you how this scenario turns out. You could just kick yourself, couldn't you?

So am I expecting you to never reward your students with something out of the ordinary? Of course not. But (don't you just love buts?) you have to build it into your policy, and I highly suggest it becomes an all or nothing policy.

Here's a suggestion of a way you could incorporate free days (or any other scenario) into your policy.

Example Policy: Students are expected to complete 50 assignments per week or 10 per day. If the entire student body has completed them in any given week and there is a period of free time, the school, at its discretion will offer a student spa day. No student's may perform spa services on each other while on the clock unless all students are approved.

So what would happen if only 90% of the student body had their assignments done? They would probably encourage the rest to hurry and get it done so that everyone could participate. What would happen if the other 10% did not finish, nobody gets a spa day.

Why all or nothing? First off, it encourages the students to hold each other accountable and stay actively engaged. Second off, students love to claim favoritism. By incorporating an all or nothing policy it avoids this nasty little scenario altogether.

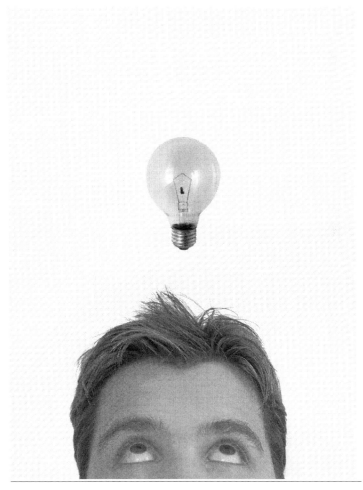

LEADERSHIP JOURNAL

_____

_____

_____

_____

_____

_____

_____

_____

_____

_____

_____

_____

_____

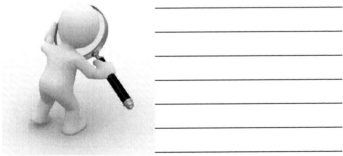

LEADERSHIP JOURNAL

_____

_____

_____

_____

_____

_____

_____

_____

_____

_____

_____

_____

_____

_____

_____

_____

_____

_____

_____

_____

_____

_____

_____

_____

_____

_____

OBSERVE

I'm not smart, but I like to observe. Millions saw the apple fall, but Newton was the one who asked why.

William Hazlitt

This piece of advice is for everyone. Owners, directors, and instructors.

You can get a lot of work done by observing. Take a few minutes each day and just walk around your school.

Don't talk, don't look for anything in particular, just observe.

Listen in on the conversations your students are having.

Notice where everyone is congregating.

Notice how your fellow instructors interact with the students, or how the students interact with the instructors.

Look at the type of client's that are in the school right now. What services are they having done? Are the services being performed well?

Look at the restrooms and the floors and the walls. Are they clean? Is there hair on the floor? Are the mirrors dirty?

Observe from a client's or potential student's perspective. What do you see?

You learn more from observing your surroundings everyday than you ever will by asking people about what's going on around you.

I read a book once on management, one of the things they talked about was a thing they called, MBWA.

This stands for: Manage By Walking Around.

So why this technique? Besides observing what's going on

around you, it lets your student's and other staff know you care.

When you're physically present in someone's life, they associate that with being emotionally present.

Remember one of the most important keys to good leadership is the ability to build deep, meaningful connections with each of your students and co-workers. You can't do that stuck behind a desk or hiding in a classroom all day.

Some of you classroom teachers may be wondering if how you're going to do this. You can't just leave your classroom can you?

Yes, being a classroom instructor does make MBWA more challenging but if you took a few minutes out of your breaks to just walk around and connect with the student's you don't see every day it will go a long way in keeping those relationships solid.

Why do we keep on talking about relationships over and over again?

Well, because if you get nothing else from this book

except for the understanding that it's important to build good relationships. You'll be a successful leader.

Remember when we talked about the beauty of managing agreements? Later we'll talk about why your student's become defensive when you manage those agreements.

If you have a personal (not home-life personal, school-life personal) relationship with every student do you think it's less likely that they will become defensive when we manage agreements with them?

If you have a close relationship with another one of your instructors do you think they would take it personally if you pointed out that they may have made a mistake?

If you have a close relationship with your manager or owner, would it make it easier for you to go to them with questions or concerns?

Take the opportunity to strengthen relationships wherever and whenever you can and you will find it makes your leadership stronger and more rewarding.

Have friends and family observe also. Each month have an instructor invite a family member or friend into the school to become a secret shopper.

Let them enjoy a complimentary service for honest feedback on the services and professionalism of the students and staff.

Bring in secret shoppers to ask about enrollment. How are they greeted, are they given a tour? How interested does your staff act when it comes to enrollment?

Take all this information back to your staff meetings and discuss it. Make goals to improve.

Give your students feedback on their secret shoppers. If you consistently bring in secret shoppers, it won't take long for your students to stay on top of their own professional behavior!

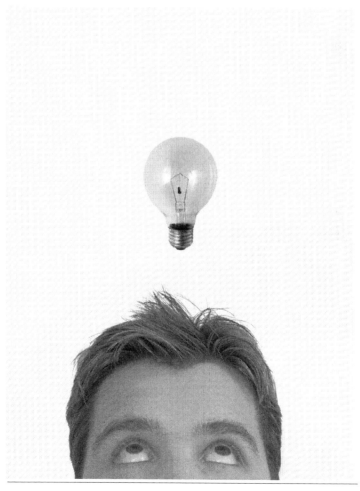

LEADERSHIP JOURNAL

LEADERSHIP JOURNAL

_____

_____

_____

_____

_____

_____

_____

_____

_____

_____

_____

_____

_____

_____

_____

_____

_____

_____

_____

_____

_____

_____

_____

_____

PLEASE AND THANK YOU.

Friends and good manners will carry you where money won't go.

Margaret Walker

Not all leadership skills have to do with directly managing students. Nor should leadership progression take place solely during school hours. To be a leader, you should practice leadership skills in multiple ways, in and out of school.

Make being a leader part of who you are as a person.

Manners are a great way to show people what type of person you are. (And that's a fantastic one!)

What do you think of when you think of good manners? Are manners something that your mother drilled into you as a child? Most think that by the time they are adults, people know what good manners are.

Of course everyone should know how to say please and thank you. And I hope that you say them without even having to think about it.

Here are some other ways that you, as a professional could and should use good manners to elevate your professional confidence.

Greeting People:

Very first and foremost you should always look people in the eye whenever you speak to them. Secondly, when meeting someone for the first time extend your arm and shake their hand.

Do you get nervous meeting people for the first time? Chances are they do too. Being the first to smile and offer a handshake shows that you are confident (even when you don't feel it). At a loss for words? Start out with something as simple as, "Hi, my name is _____, how are you today?

Pay attention when someone offers you their name. People love the sound of their own name. Try to use it once or twice in the conversation. This lets them know you are connected to them and it helps you to remember.

The best conversations to have with potential connections are about them, ask lots of questions. If you find your conversation slipping, here's a few great conversation starters you can try.

I love your name, what does it mean? (If they have an unusual name)

Where are you from?

Where did you go to school?

What made you decide to become a (profession)?

Did you hear about (current event)?

Have you ever met (name of person in your business circle)?

You remind me of (celebrity or mutual friend).

Remember, even when you're not in the office or school, you will still have the opportunity to meet new and interesting people. Smile and make eye contact with people in the grocery store, in the theatre line or in a restaurant. These make good practice opportunities on being able to start and carry on a conversations with people you've just met.

Make it a goal to start three conversations this week. Record your results on your journal page.

Practice Putting Others First:

Open the door for people. Yes, anyone, man, woman, child, elder, or tattooed punk.

Let someone with less items cut ahead of you in line.

Shovel your neighbor's sidewalk.

Hold your tongue when fighting with your spouse.

By getting in the habit of putting others first, it literally changes you and everything else around you. This may sound far-fetched or slightly hokey-pokey but give it a try. Go out of your way to look for opportunities to help others. I promise by doing this it will increase your self-confidence. When our confidence increases you'll find you feel like Superman or Wonder Woman. Other concepts in this book will seem easier with your newfound super powers. Do you believe in the law of Karma? I do. Put good and positive deeds out there and watch them come back to you ten-fold. Don't forget to journal your results!

Cell Phone Etiquette:

Cell phones have become an extension of our hands. Notice people around you, how close is their cell phone to them? Within arm's reach for sure. No wonder our students can't be without them.

What do you do when your phone rings or buzzes with a text? You probably can't help but look at it. Even in the middle of a conversation with someone else. We don't think twice about putting our face-to-face conversations on hold to answer our phones. We even go as far as "discreetly" texting under our desks or tables while in meetings.

People need to feel important. That's why we text and

answer calls at inappropriate times. Because it makes us feel important. But as a leader, remember your job is to make *other* people feel important. How do we do this in this age of technology? It's as simple as putting your phone on silent and away during conversations with other people. Don't even be tempted.

Bottom line- looking at or responding to cell phone texts and calls in meetings is rude. Don't do it.

Emails and Phone Messages:

Remember our chapter on Juggling is for Clowns? We talked about making a to-do list and knocking them out in order of importance?

Messages, emails, notes and other inquiries should always be number one in your day. There is nothing worse than sending out an email or leaving a message and having to wait for a reply. Remember, other's time is just as valuable as your own. By replying in a timely manner, it lets people know you find them valuable and that you can be depended on. Two very important traits in any business.

Make a commitment that you will answer all messages

within 24 hours.

Practice Punctuality:

Are you always on time to work and other scheduled events? How often do you call in sick, take long lunches or schedule your doctor appointments during your work day?

Again, this goes back to being dependable. If people know they can depend on you to show up, they know they can depend on you for other things too.

Practice Good Grooming and Hygiene:

First impressions count. Second impressions count too. People see how you take care of yourself and your surroundings and make assumptions about how you take care of business. Would you hire you based on today's appearance?

The Power of a Positive Attitude

Most people don't think of having a positive attitude as a good manner, but I beg to differ. This good manner tip may even seem a bit cliché to you, and that's okay. But it's still every bit as important. As a matter of fact, without a positive attitude it's really hard to have good manners. Believe it or not, having a positive attitude is very hard for a lot of people. You may be one of them. Do you see the glass as half empty, or half full?

If you have been exhibiting a negative attitude and expecting failure and difficulties, now is the time to change the way you think. It's time to get rid of negative thoughts and behavior and lead a happier and more successful life. If you have tried and failed, it only means that you have not tried enough. Her are a few tips that may help you develop a more positive attitude.

1. Choose to be happy. Yes, this is your life and you have a choice.

2. Associate yourself with happy people. Avoid those that spread gossip and breed negativity. (Acknowledge this may be you, and you owe it to yourself and others around you to stop.)

3. Read inspiring stories or watch uplifting movies.

4. Pick out some quotes that inspire you and post

them where you can see them every day. Share them with others.

5. Repeat affirmations that motivate you.

6. Visualize yourself as a positive person. Visualize happy endings where you normally see failures.

7. Practice, Practice, Practice.

Becoming more positive takes dedication and repeat performances. If you find yourself feeling negative, acknowledge that it's okay, you're human after all. Remind yourself of your progress and keep moving forward.

Just like riding a bike, the more you practice being positive, the easier it will become.

Last But Not Least:

Please and thank you are two (actually, three) of the most important words in the English language. Use them.

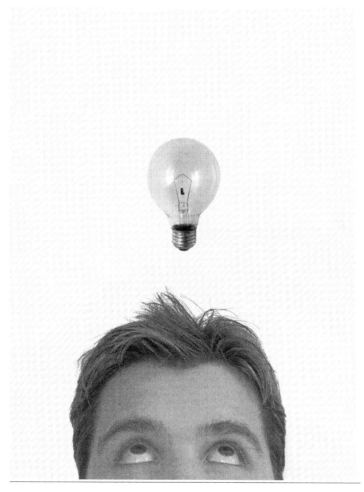

147

LEADERSHIP JOURNAL

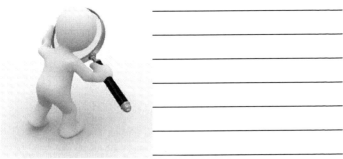

LEADERSHIP JOURNAL

QUESTION EVERYTHING.

Don't Make Assumptions. Find the courage to ask questions and to express what you really want. Communicate with others as clearly as you can to avoid misunderstandings, sadness and drama. With just this one agreement, you can completely transform your life.

Miguel Angel Ruiz

One of my favorite books in all the world is, The Four Agreements, by Don Miguel Ruiz. If you're looking for a life changing book, that's got to be the one!

In that book he talks about how we as a society make a lot of assumptions. We take these assumptions as fact and build our world around them.

I'm going to use my good old friend Phil Collins as a perfect example of this. (Now, before you go making an assumption and want me to arrange a meeting with him. I need to clarify, we are not actually friends.)

Most people have heard his song, "In the Air Tonight". Have you heard this song? It's simply amazing! Google the song right now if you haven't- you're in for a treat.

According to the majority of Phil Collin's fans that song was actually written about an incident in Phil's life.

You may have heard a story similar to this one.

"The story has to do with Phil Collins supposedly watching his close friend drown from a nearby cliff, while he stood helpless, too far away to rescue. In addition, supposedly there was a man who could have rescued the friend but just stood idly by. Then, Phil writes a song about the experience and gives the man a front row ticket to the show where he premieres the song. While Phil sings the song to him, the spotlight is on the man in the front row."

You go Phil!

Way to show him!

Now I hate to be the bearer of bad news, but this story is false. Here's what Phil Collins had to say about the story.

"I don't know what this song is about. When I was writing this I was going through a divorce. And the only thing I can say about it is that it's obviously in anger. It's the angry side, or the bitter side of a separation. So what makes it even more comical is when I hear these stories which started many years ago, particularly in America, of someone come up to me and say, 'Did you really see someone drowning?' I said, 'No, wrong'. And then every time I go back to America the story gets Chinese whispers, it gets more and more elaborate. It's so frustrating, 'cos this is one song out of all the songs probably that I've ever written that I really don't know what it's about, you know." -Phil Collins, via BBC Worldwide

Mystery solved. Thanks Phil.

Another example would be to look at the tabloids every day in the supermarket. If those celebrities were pregnant every time we read that they were we would need to build a whole new state of California just to shelter all those cute little celebri-tots

How many times have you based decisions around information you later found out was false.

As a leader, you make lots of important decisions every day. It's important that you base them on truth and fact.

Next time someone gossips or gives you information, instead of taking them at their word. Make a commitment to investigate.

You need to be a seeker of truth for yourself, your school, and your students!

This is a good point to take back to your students. When they come and ask questions. Have them seek out the answers and share them with you.

OWNERS/DIRECTORS:

Chances are you have an instructor or staff member on board right now who likes to fill you in on the staff gossip. Take the time right now to think of each one of your staff members. What are your beliefs about them? Where did these beliefs come from?

Chances are you're missing out on developing some great relationships with your staff members because you're holding back on assumptions and untruths.

YOU need to develop a personal relationship with each and every staff member. YOU need to be comfortable enough to go to them for clarification on anything.

If your staff members do not feel comfortable coming and speaking with you openly and honestly, you need to find out why. Read the chapter on surrendering your ego and get to work strengthening your team.

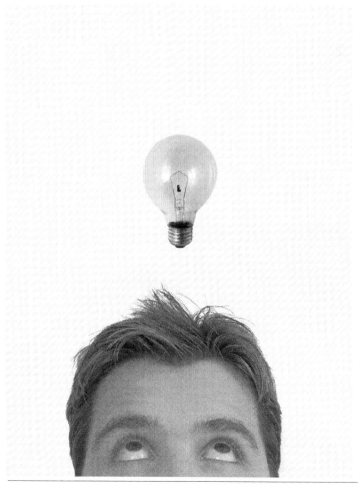

LEADERSHIP JOURNAL

_____

_____

_____

_____

_____

_____

_____

_____

_____

_____

_____

_____

_____

_____

_____

_____

_____

_____

_____

_____

_____

_____

LEADERSHIP JOURNAL

REMOVE *YOURSELF* FROM THE SITUATION

Respect your efforts, respect yourself. Self-respect leads to self-discipline.
When you have both firmly under your belt, that's real power.

Clint Eastwood

This was one of the best pieces of advice I've ever received as a school director and educator and I can't wait to share it with you.

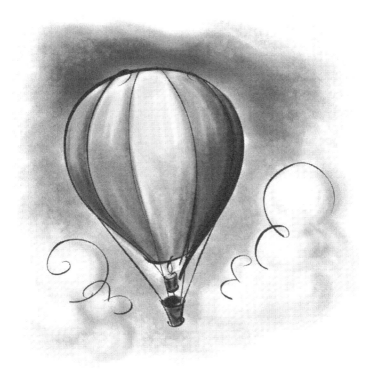

See that balloon on the top of the page? That's you! No, I'm not saying you're full of hot air. I'm saying that if you look at things from a different perspective it can make all the difference in the world.

Think of a situation that you're battling right now. Or maybe one you've battled in the past, but can't seem to move past it. How do you feel when you think about it? Embarrassed, Annoyed? Angry? Defensive? Bitter?

Now, remove _YOURSELF_ from the situation. Things seem a lot worse than they are when we let our emotions tell the story.

How?

Step one: Look at the issue objectively. Take your emotions out of it by imagining it didn't happen to you, or that you're telling the story of someone else. What if this scenario were happening to a friend or co-worker. Would you think the situation was so terrible? What advice would you give them? Probably to stop worrying so much and to move on. Now, give yourself that same advice.

Step two: Be the balloon. Picture yourself above the situation. Look at the big picture as a whole. Look at your end goal. See how small the problem is when your way up there looking down? Now how big is the problem? In the big scheme of things? Probably not so big.

The key is to give yourself permission to feel those emotions of embarrassment, annoyance, anger, and defensiveness. When you allow yourself to feel, you grow. Now, give yourself permission to let it go and heal. It's only when you heal that you progress.

LEADERSHIP JOURNAL

LEADERSHIP JOURNAL

S

SURRENDER YOUR EGO

I work really hard at trying to see the big picture and not getting stuck in ego. I believe we're all put on this planet for a purpose, and we all have a different purpose... When you connect with that love and that compassion, that's when everything unfolds.

Ellen DeGeneres

We've been talking a lot about how to increase confidence. And confidence is good in leadership. As a matter of fact, confidence is a must in order to be a great leader. You need to believe in yourself and your capabilities in order to be successful.

So what does it mean when I say surrender your ego?

Well, it means that part of this whole leadership process is going to hurt. How?

You're going to discover you're not perfect! Congratulations!

You're probably thinking right now, "Duh, I know I'm not perfect."

But this chapter is not really about realizing you're not perfect, it's about what we do when we realize we're not perfect. When we realize that we've made a mistake.

You may have even done it without thinking when I mentioned your imperfection.

We become *DEFENSIVE!*

We feel we have to justify why we did this or thought this, or acted upon this.

We cannot sit in our own imperfection and say to ourselves or another, "Well, looks like a screwed that up!" No, it's easier to blame it on something or someone else.

Other people do it when we call them out on their imperfections, suddenly, they didn't know it wasn't right, it wasn't their idea, and it wasn't their fault!

Take any scenario you've ever had with any student and you'll find this to be true.

They make a mistake or get caught breaking a policy, let's say dress code for instance. Suddenly *you* must have changed the dress code, they had no idea they couldn't wear that. They've seen other students wear that and no one sent *them* home. The nerve of you and the school for singling them out! Sound familiar?

When was the last time you had a student just say, "You're right, I knew it, I tried to get away with it. I'll clock out and go change right now." If this has happened you need to figure out how to clone them and send them my way.

Have you ever had a friend, or co-worker, or boss, or student just fess up and tell you they made a mistake. No arguments, no excuses?

What did you do? What did you think?

I always feel quick to forgive someone who fesses up. I respect a person who confesses to making mistakes. It makes me feel that it is okay for me to make mistakes also, and heaven knows I do it often and well.

So next time you make a mistake, surrender your ego and admit it. No excuses. See? Doesn't that feel good?

One more important note on this topic-

Sometimes ego gets in the way when acknowledging other's work. If your co-worker, instructor or student comes up with a great idea, tell everyone whose great idea it was.

Everyone deserves to be acknowledged for their contributions to your success.

It doesn't take anything away from you when you give compliments freely to others.

LEADERSHIP JOURNAL

LEADERSHIP JOURNAL

_____

_____

_____

_____

_____

_____

_____

_____

_____

_____

_____

_____

_____

_____

_____

_____

_____

_____

_____

_____

_____

_____

TRY AGAIN.

If at first you don't succeed, try, try again. Then quit. There's no point in being a damn fool about it.

W. C. Fields

This chapter is short and sweet and needs no further explanation.

Never give up on the person you are meant to be.

Every day is a new day, with no mistakes in it.

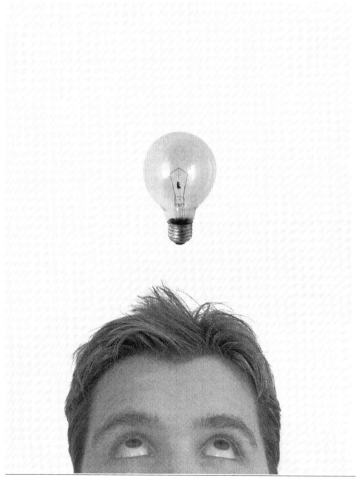

LEADERSHIP JOURNAL

_____

_____

_____

_____

_____

_____

_____

_____

_____

_____

_____

_____

_____

_____

_____

_____

_____

_____

_____

_____

LEADERSHIP JOURNAL

_____

_____

_____

_____

_____

_____

_____

_____

_____

_____

_____

_____

_____

_____

_____

_____

_____

_____

_____

_____

_____

_____

_____

_____

_____

_____

U

UNDERSTAND NOTHING.

Information is not knowledge.

Albert Einstein

V

VALUE EVERYTHING.

What is a cynic? A man who knows the price of everything and the value of nothing.

Oscar Wilde

Why did I put these two chapters together? Because they belong together.

Life works in mysterious ways. Your life has a distinct pattern and purpose to it. Have you ever taken a moment to think about that? Everything you've done has led you up to this point right now. And right here is where you are meant to be. You matter. Whether you like it or not, the things you will do and say every day of your life will have an impact on your future self, and the lives of those around you. Decisions you make now and in the future will lead you on this crazy journey that is your life.

Becoming the leader and person you want to be is a life-long endeavor. As you look back you'll be able to see how the days and moments add up to make the greater whole, and how each moment counted.

Live in every moment, good or bad. You don't have to understand and make sense of everything. But you should value everything.

Appreciate the fact that you're a part of an amazing industry. That you've been given the opportunity to change people's lives. That's a big responsibility!

It's going to be important on those really hard days to remember that you have a choice, and you have chosen to make a difference.

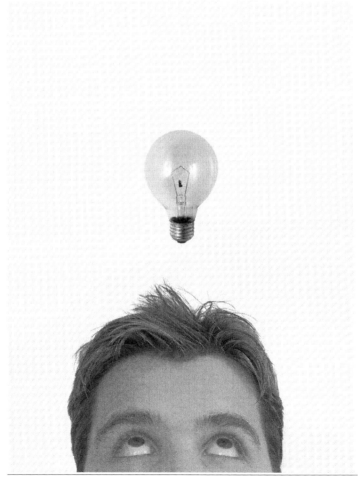

LEADERSHIP JOURNAL

LEADERSHIP JOURNAL

WRITE IT DOWN OR IT DIDN'T HAPPEN

What is a diary as a rule? A document useful to the person who keeps it. Dull to the contemporary who reads it and invaluable to the student, centuries afterwards, who treasures it.

Walter Scott

Everything you do and say should be documented. Wait, what?

Let's start with our students. Every meeting you have with every student should be documented in some form of a communication log.

Suggestion: Use a large three ring binder and tabs and separate it by student. Make a standard communication form and have every staff member fill one out when meeting with students. For clarification, I'm not suggesting filling out a form every time you say hello to a student. Use these for, "Hey, I'm asking you to please put your cell phone away." Or yes, I have time to go over your hours or goals, here's what we came up with."

These documents are not intended for disciplinary forms, although they could be. They are a way of documenting a student's history, good or bad.

What's so great about it? Well if I'm an instructor who sees the phone out and I think I'm giving them their first warning and I grab the binder and see they've already been told once today, guess what I'm going to do? I'm going to document it again, but I'm also going to give them a disciplinary write up.

Sometimes, we get busy or just forget to communicate with our fellow instructors what actions or words we've used that day.

Let's go back to the chapter where we talked about consistency. This is another method you can use to nip that chatter.

When we have students that exhibit bad behavior, a lot of times they have gotten away with it for a long period of time. Why? Because each instructor may believe that the student has been warned once, but if every instructor gives them a warning they've received five warnings. You better believe the other students see it to.

How many times have you or your school given out verbal warnings that never amount to anything? And we wonder why we have no control over our student's or our school. Things must be documented. Everything should be documented.

Use that documentation when you sit down with your student and manage agreements.

Picture your school like a court of law. Documentation is proof of an event. What would happen if you went to court without proof? They would throw out your case.

Another thing to consider when documenting is that you should only document behavior that you have seen yourself. If another student comes up to you and says, "I saw Suzie drinking in the parking lot." Guess what, it didn't happen. Now if that student is willing to document and sign stating that they saw Susie drinking in the parking lot, then that's another story

Another reason why documentation is important? When your accrediting agencies come in, they are a government appointed agency. They are their own court of law. They are your court of law. You need documentation of every action you've taken against every student.

What else should you document? Staff meetings, advisory meetings and industry meetings.

Keeping records is just good business. It will also serve as a professional journal. You can look back at times when completion or moral was high or low and see what you were doing differently.

SCHOOL DIRECTORS/OWNERS:

You spend countless hours poring over government standards and policies. I know you tell your staff over and over again how important it is that they document everything. But do you explain why?

Sometimes we get in the habit of saying, this is my job and this is your job. I'll do mine and you do yours. But this is a mistake.

Get your staff involved in learning a little about accreditation and DOE requirements. They will come to understand the importance of documenting. And how much work it takes "behind the scenes" to run a school

On the other side of the coin. How long has it been since you were "out in the trenches"? Recognize that they have a hard job too.

Ask them questions. Seek their advice and counsel. Believe me, most of the time they have a much clearer picture of what's going on in your school than you do.

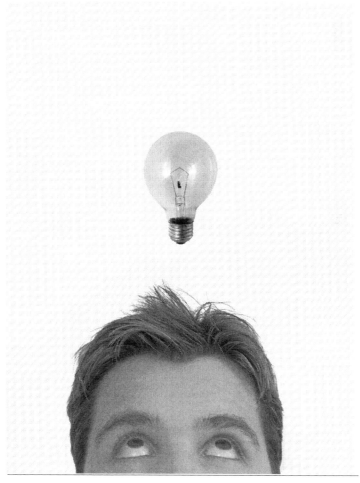

LEADERSHIP JOURNAL

LEADERSHIP JOURNAL

X MARKS THE SPOT

"No thief, however skillful, can rob one of knowledge, and that is why knowledge is the best and safest treasure to acquire."

—L. Frank Baum,

Looks like we're nearing the end of our journey. Now is a great time to revisit the steps you've taken to become a better leader. Use this chapter as a review tool and checklist. What are you doing well at this point? What could you be working on?

You may have even made some of your own goals during this time, how are those developing?

Remember, practice makes progress, before it makes perfect.

Remind yourself why you decided to become an educator.

Know and understand your school's policies. Know and understand your student handbook.

Have knowledge of how your government agencies work and how they affect you.

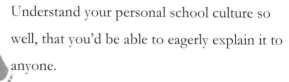

Don't wait for information to be given to you. Research and gather information without prompting.

Consider first, believe in, carryout, and be loyal to the established objectives of your institution.

Understand your personal school culture so well, that you'd be able to eagerly explain it to anyone.

Elevate yourself so that **all** the staff is working as one united entity. Put your relationships with your school staff before anything else.

 Work together and reinforce each other.

Build a solid curriculum for your students and show them what it takes to be successful.

 Fill the "future boss" role and demonstrate to your students how to develop a professional working relationship. Keep on your side of the no friend zone.

 Manage by walking around.

Stay organized. Get your daily duties done right away, including answering emails and retuning messages. Schedule staff coverage so that everyone has the time they need.

Practice good manners in and out of school.

 Don't make assumptions, always seek the truth for yourself.

Be fair and consistent in your actions, tone, and body language when dealing with others.

 Remove your emotions from your daily battles and choose your battles carefully.

Admit when you've made a mistake. Don't make excuses.

 Acknowledge the good work of others.

Seek out continuing education and take it back to your tribe.

 Build a vast network with other professionals, and continually develop it.

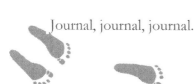 Use integrity as your main form of professional currency.

Document, document, document.

Journal, journal, journal.

 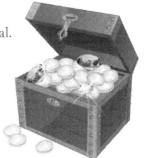

LEADERSHIP JOURNAL

LEADERSHIP JOURNAL

WHY AM I DOING THIS AGAIN?

Our deepest fear is not that we are inadequate. Our deepest fear is that we are powerful beyond measure. It is our light, not our darkness that most frightens us. We ask ourselves, who am I to be brilliant, gorgeous, talented, and fabulous? Actually, who are you not to be? You are a child of God. Your playing small does not serve the world. There is nothing enlightened about shrinking so that other people will not feel insecure around you. We are all meant to shine, as children do. We were born to make manifest the glory of God that is within us. It is not just in some of us; it is in everyone and as we let our own light shine, we unconsciously give others permission to do the same. As we are liberated from our own fear, our presence automatically liberates others.

Marianne Williamson

Do you still feel like an imposter? Maybe so. Hopefully less than when you began this journey. Remember. You have everything in you to be the person and the leader you want to be.

Your school has the potential of turning out the best of

what this industry has to offer in the coming years and decades. How does it feel to say that you are a part of shaping our future generations of hairdressers? Hairdressers, who are a part of shaping trends? Future trends are what shape ideas, and what shape people.

You are contributing to our world in a unique way,

The question is, how much you are willing to contribute? Remember, it starts with you. It starts with your co-workers, and directors and owners. It starts with your school.

We need to continually strive for excellence so that we can give the best of who we are to our students.

This journey does not end with the final chapter in this book. It will indeed be a lifelong journey.

I would like to personally invite anyone to reach out to me at any time. Let me be part of your support.

Oh, and I love success stories. If any part of this book touched you or helped you, please email and let me know.

christa@emmceedee.com

LEADERSHIP JOURNAL

LEADERSHIP JOURNAL

_____

_____

_____

_____

_____

_____

_____

_____

_____

_____

_____

_____

_____

_____

_____

_____

_____

_____

_____

_____

_____

_____

_____

_____

_____

Z

ZEN. FIND YOUR PEACE AT THE END OF EACH DAY.

"Learning to let go should be learned before learning to get. Life should be touched, not strangled. You've got to relax, let it happen at times, and at others move forward with it."
— Ray Bradbury

The day is over. It's now time to let those worries slip away for a few hours. Don't forget, the best leaders know how to balance home and work.

Rest, renew and be ready to go at it again tomorrow.

Included in this chapter are a few of my favorite quotes, which motivate and inspire me. I hope they offer you a little Zen too. Enjoy!

Nothing is impossible, the word itself says 'I'm possible'!
Audrey Hepburn

I hated every minute of training, but I said, 'Don't quit. Suffer now and live the rest of your life as a champion.'
Muhammad Ali

Thousands of candles can be lighted from a single candle, and the life of the candle will not be shortened. Happiness never decreases by being shared.
Buddha

We must let go of the life we have planned, so as to accept the one that is waiting for us.
Joseph Campbell

Try to be a rainbow in someone's cloud.
Maya Angelou

What lies behind you and what lies in front of you, pales in comparison to what lies inside of you.
Ralph Waldo Emerson

It is never too late to be what you might have been.
George Eliot

I believe that one defines oneself by reinvention. To not be like your parents. To not be like your friends. To be yourself. To cut yourself out of stone.

Henry Rollins

Tomorrow is the most important thing in life. Comes into us at midnight very clean. It's perfect when it arrives and it puts itself in our hands. It hopes we've learned something from yesterday.

John Wayne

If we did all the things we are capable of, we would literally astound ourselves.

Thomas A. Edison

Everyone has inside of him a piece of good news. The good news is that you don't know how great you can be! How much you can love! What you can accomplish! And what your potential is!

Anne Frank

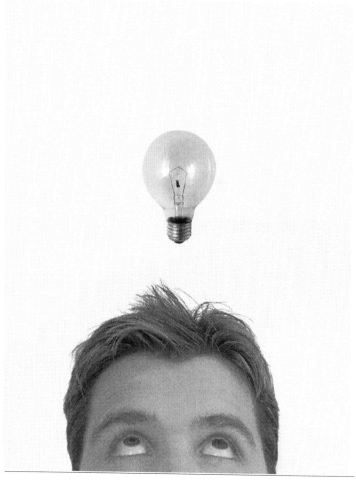

LEADERSHIP JOURNAL

LEADERSHIP JOURNAL

_____

_____

_____

_____

_____

_____

_____

_____

_____

_____

_____

_____

_____

_____

_____

_____

_____

_____

_____

_____

_____

_____

_____

_____

ABOUT THE AUTHOR

Christa McDearmon is a licensed Cosmetologist, Barber, Master Esthetician and Instructor. She began her career 18 years ago in Las Vegas, Nevada.

She has since had many incredible opportunities presented to her due to her hard work and professional dedication. Including becoming an Industry Educator, Instructor, Educational Director, Cosmetology School Manager, and Author, all while consistently working behind the chair.

Through all of these wonderful opportunities Christa discovered that educating others was her true purpose and passion, she dreamed of one day being able to open a company that focused on continuing education and professional growth. In 2013, with the help of many mentors, industry friends, and the support of outstanding educational companies, Emmceedee Education, LLC was born.

She currently resides in Janesville, WI with her husband Brian, and son Nolan.

Christa can be contacted at Christa@Emmceedee.com.

Made in the USA
Monee, IL
05 October 2021